Alternative Treatments of Dementia and Mild Cognitive Impairment

Safe, effective and affordable approaches and how to use them

James Lake, MD

© 2015 James H. Lake

All rights reserved. First published in 2015 under the title "Dementia and Mild Cognitive Impairment (MCI): The Integrative Mental Health Solution," revised and re-published in 2019. This book contains material protected under International and Federal Copyright Laws and Treaties. Any unauthorized reprint or use of this material is prohibited. No part of this book may be reproduced or transmitted in any form or by any means, electronic or mechanical, including photocopying, recording, or by any information storage or retrieval system without express written permission from the author/publisher. Copyright protection of the cover image 'the eye of the flower,' by Nicole Asselborn, MD, is included under the above provisions.

This book is dedicated to my best friend and soul mate, Nicole Asselborn, MD, with gratitude for invaluable advice on the right scope and voice for this project, and for coming up with the lovely image on the cover.

Contents

Part I: Introduction

- What this book is about
- How to use this book
- Alternative and integrative medicine defined
- Integrative mental health care defined
- About Dr. Lake's background and qualifications
- What to do if you—or someone you are caring for—have severe symptoms of cognitive impairment

Part II: Understanding and treating mild cognitive impairment (MCI), Alzheimer's disease and other forms of dementia from a holistic point of view

- MCI, Alzheimer's disease and other forms of dementia—overview
- Taking inventory of your symptoms
- Identifying treatments that make sense for you: evaluating the evidence
- Alternative treatments of MCI, Alzheimer's disease and other forms of dementia
- Developing a treatment plan that is *appropriate for you or a person you are caring for*
- Making changes along the way: re-evaluating the treatment plan and making it better
- Repeating the steps until you find a treatment plan that *works for you*

- Summary of main points

Going deeper

Finding quality products and services on the internet

Disclaimer

The information in this book is intended to provide information on the treatment of mild cognitive impairment (MCI), Alzheimer's disease and other forms of dementia, and does not constitute medical advice. The publisher and author are not responsible for any specific health needs that may require medical supervision, and are not liable for any damages or negative consequences from any treatment, action or application to any person reading or using the information in this book. References to internet resources are provided for informational purposes only and do not constitute endorsement of any websites or other sources. Readers should be aware that the websites listed in this book may change.

Part I: Introduction

What this book is about

My chief goal in writing this book and the others in the series was to create a practical low-cost resource on safe and effective alternative treatments of mental health problems including herbals, vitamins and other natural supplements, mind-body approaches, and energy therapies.

The subject of this book is mild cognitive impairment (MCI) and dementia. You will learn about a variety of safe and effective alternative treatments of MCI and dementia. If you—or someone you are caring for—are struggling with memory loss, confusion, or another cognitive problem that is interfering with your ability to perform daily activities, or if you are taking a medication that isn't helping, this book provides valuable information about alternative treatments of MCI and dementia and practical strategies for how to use them.

If you've experienced memory loss, confusion or other cognitive problems in the past and you are now functioning better, this book will help you create a wellness plan that fits your lifestyle. By the time you finish reading you'll be able to create an individualized care plan adapted to your needs, preferences and budget. Just as important, you will learn how to *think about* your mental health care in a more holistic way.

How to use this book

This book was *written to give you the maximum amount of information in the least amount of time*. The last section of each book is a summary of the most important points. I've provided links to valuable internet resources to help you find quality brands of natural supplements and other alternative treatments, important safety information and professional help if you think you need it.

If you are a mental health professional this book provides concise, jargon-free summaries of scientifically validated alternative treatments you can use when advising clients about safe, effective alternative treatments of mild cognitive impairment (MCI) and Alzheimer's disease or other forms of dementia.

Alternative and integrative medicine defined

Alternative medicine—sometimes called 'complementary and alternative medicine or CAM—consists of approaches that are currently not used in mainstream Western medicine (also called 'biomedicine' and 'allopathic medicine'). Examples of CAM include acupuncture, herbs and other natural supplements, so-called 'energy' therapies such as Healing Touch, and others.

Integrative medicine is a rapidly growing model of care that takes a middle ground between Western medicine as conventionally practiced and CAM. Integrative medicine:

- is a person-centered approach

- that takes account of the needs and preferences of each unique person

- that focuses on maintaining optimal health and treating symptoms

- uses both conventional mainstream approaches like medications and psychotherapy, and complementary and alternative (CAM) therapies like herbal medicines and acupuncture

- is based on the *best available* scientific evidence

Integrative mental health care defined

Integrative mental health care is a specialized area of integrative medicine aimed at helping each person find safe, appropriate and effective treatments for their mental health problem taking into account their unique symptoms, values, preferences and circumstances.

Integrative mental health care often includes advice on life-style changes that require on-going commitment to improving health and mental health such as changing your diet, exercising more, sleeping better, and using relaxation techniques to reduce stress. In addition to lifestyle changes integrative mental health care may include advice on select herbals, vitamins and other natural supplements when there is evidence for both their safety and effectiveness. Finally, Integrative mental health care may include prescription medications or other conventionally used treatments.

If this is the first time you've heard about integrative mental health care and want to find out more before trying a new treatment for anxiety, I encourage you to download the [first book in the series](#) to learn more. This book is available as a free download and will give you an overview of essential concepts and methods in integrative mental health care.

About Dr. Lake's background and qualifications

I completed my medical training at University of California, Irvine, and did my residency in adult psychiatry at Stanford University Hospital. I am board-certified by the American Board of Psychiatry and Neurology, and I have practiced psychiatry for more than 20 years in diverse settings. I've had extensive experience taking care of patients in hospitals, clinics, emergency rooms and in my private practice. I have been a student of herbal medicine for decades and I am certified in medical acupuncture and in EEG biofeedback. I previously served on the teaching faculty at Stanford University Hospital and I am currently an adjunct clinical assistant professor in the Department of Psychiatry at University of Arizona College of Medicine. I've taught physicians and other mental health professionals about integrative mental healthcare at national and international conferences. I publish a column on integrative mental health care in *Psychiatric Times,* a leading trade publication for mental health professionals and I am a frequent blogger on Psychology Today. I've authored numerous articles and chapters in medical journals and textbooks, and I've written, co-authored or edited five textbooks covering the philosophy, theory and practice of integrative mental healthcare.

I've been involved in national and international efforts to establish integrative mental healthcare as a new medical sub-specialty in its own right. I founded and previously chaired an initiative aimed at changing mental health care into a more effective, safer and more person-centered model of care: the American Psychiatric Association Caucus on Complementary and Integrative Medicine. An important goal of the Caucus is the development of expert resources for educating and training psychiatrists in the safe, *evidence-based* uses of non-medication treatments for treating anxiety, depression and the other common mental health problems covered in the book series.

What to do if you—or someone you are caring for—have severe symptoms of cognitive impairment

Severe symptoms of cognitive impairment that often occur in Alzheimer's disease and other forms of dementia include:

- Inability to recall recent or remote events
- Difficulty understanding spoken or written language
- Getting lost in familiar places
- Not recognizing people who you know
- Getting confused about the time of day, date or season
- Loss of the ability to perform routine daily tasks

If you have one or more severe problems affecting your memory or cognition you probably need more help than this short book can provide. ***If you—or someone you are caring for—are impaired by severe memory loss, confusion, or other severe cognitive symptoms, I encourage you to consult with a psychiatrist or other mental health provider.***

Part II: Understanding and treating mild cognitive impairment (MCI), Alzheimer's disease and other forms of dementia from a holistic point of view

MCI, Alzheimer's disease and other forms of dementia: overview

The information in the following sections will help you better understand Alzheimer's disease and less severe forms of cognitive impairment, and give you tools you need to develop a safe and affordable treatment plan.

Dementia

Dementia is a chronic condition characterized by severe persisting impairments of short-term and long-term memory and severe deficits in other areas of cognitive functioning such as abstract reasoning, language, impaired capacity to perform routine daily tasks, and loss of ability to recognize familiar objects, places or people.

Medical causes of dementia include vascular disease that affects the arteries of the brain (*vascular dementia*), Parkinson's disease, other neurodegenerative disorders, traumatic brain injury (TBI), HIV/AIDS, severe cerebrovascular accidents (i.e. stroke), and the cumulative toxic effects of chronic alcohol or substance abuse.

Alzheimer's disease, the most common form of dementia, is a progressive neurodegenerative disease that accounts for two thirds of all cases of dementia. It has been estimated that roughly one half of all individuals over the age of 85 have Alzheimer's disease. Genetic risk factors, chronic nutrient deficiencies, toxic injury to the brain, coronary artery disease, chronic stress and prolonged social isolation or restricted intellectual activity increase the risk of Alzheimer's disease. The degenerative changes in the brain that lead to Alzheimer's disease are related to deposits of an abnormal brain protein called amyloid-beta which sets off wide-spread inflammation and the formation of free radicals that damage or destroy neurons.

It is important to distinguish the progressive and irreversible changes seen in Alzheimer's disease, vascular dementia, and other forms of dementia from the temporary and reversible changes in cognition associated with a state of acute confusion called *delirium*. Serious medical illnesses or acute intoxication with alcohol or drugs often manifest as delirium in which cognitive functioning is grossly impaired. Successful treatment of the underlying cause or causes of delirium restores the brain to its healthy state and cognitive functioning rapidly returns to normal.

Anyone experiencing rapidly progressing decline in cognitive functioning should be referred urgently to the nearest hospital emergency room to rule out medical causes.

Mild cognitive impairment (MCI)

Mild cognitive impairment (MCI) is a less severe form of cognitive impairment that is often temporary but may eventually progress to Alzheimer's disease or other forms of dementia. MCI sometimes takes place with normal aging, chronic nutritional deficiencies, less severe strokes, thyroid disease, and chronic alcohol or narcotic abuse. Correcting the underlying medical cause or causes of MCI usually results in rapid improvement in cognitive functioning.

Many individuals experience moderate to severe cognitive impairment as an indirect result of mental health problems, including severe depressed mood, anxiety, bipolar disorder, psychosis, chronic sleep deprivation, and chronic alcohol or drug abuse. The successful treatment of an underlying mental health problem that is impairing cognitive functioning often results in return of normal cognitive functioning.

In addition to psychological causes of cognitive impairment, a large number of medical problems such as poorly controlled diabetes, disorders of the thyroid, cancer (or side effects of chemotherapy), endocrinologic and metabolic disorders, can cause temporary disruption of normal cognitive functioning manifesting as memory loss, confusion and other cognitive problems. The type and severity of cognitive symptoms are related to the underlying causes of disruption of healthy brain function. In most cases proper treatment results in rapid return of normal cognitive functioning. However, recent studies suggest that approximately one third of individuals diagnosed with MCI eventually progress to full-blown dementia.

Taking inventory of your symptoms

This section will help you understand your symptoms of memory loss or other cognitive problems you are experiencing, and determine how severe they are. Let's start by defining what the word *symptom* means. A *symptom is something you experience inside that you can't see.* It's a subjective experience of distress that can point to a medical or mental health problem. When different symptoms occur together, they make up a particular mental health problem or *disorder*.

While many individuals who experience symptoms of mild cognitive impairment (MCI), Alzheimer's disease or other forms of dementia have similar symptoms, each person's symptoms are related to their *unique* genetic and biological constitution, social and family history, cultural and spiritual beliefs, and personal circumstances. Memory loss or other cognitive problems may be mild, moderate or severe depending on how much distress they cause and how much they interfere with your ability to function in day to day activities.

Taking inventory of your symptoms involves filling in a symptom check-list or answering several standardized questions. Going through this process will give you important insights that will help you develop a treatment plan based on your particular symptoms of memory loss, confusion or other problems with executive functioning. If you are reading the e-book you can click here to get to psychological assessment tools that you can use to evaluate your symptoms of memory loss and the other mental health problems covered in this series of books. If you are reading the print book you can find on-line psychological assessment tools at http://www.theintegrativementalhealthsolution.com/self-assesment-questionaires.html.

If you are experiencing memory problems or other cognitive problems, I encourage you to ask someone you trust to help you answer the standardized questions in order to get a more accurate picture of your symptoms. Remember to keep a record of your results so that you can track changes in your symptoms over time. I encourage you to take inventory frequently in order to find out how well your symptoms are responding to treatment. You can use the results to optimize your current treatment plan or develop a completely new treatment plan.

If you are experiencing memory loss or other symptoms of cognitive impairment together with depressed mood, mood swings, anxiety, or another mental health problem I encourage you to complete the assessment test for that problem also. *If you are severely depressed and contemplating suicide please seek emergency care as soon as possible.*

Identifying treatments that make sense for you: evaluating the evidence

This section provides concise reviews of the evidence for a variety of alternative approaches to MCI and dementia. In addition to select natural supplements, other alternative approaches that are sometimes beneficial for symptoms of MCI, Alzheimer's disease and other forms of dementia include dietary changes, exercise, transcranial electrical stimulation and the Bredesen protocol.

Natural supplements used to treat MCI and dementia include *Ginkgo biloba*, idebenone, huperzine, some compound herbal formulas and the amino acid acetyl-l-carnitine. The majority of herbals and other natural supplements have few or mild adverse effects when a quality brand is used at the recommended dosage. However, some natural supplements can cause serious side effects when taken at inappropriate high dosages or in combination with medications. *Please read the comments on safety before trying any herbal or other natural supplement.*

The various alternative treatments of MCI and dementia can be divided into 5 categories:

- **Biological treatments** have beneficial effects at the level of a well-defined molecular mechanism. Natural supplements work in this way.

- **Whole body approaches** have general beneficial effects on the body as a whole, improve both physical and mental health and enhance well-being. Exercise and massage are examples of whole-body approaches.

- **Mindfulness and mind-body approaches** are based on concepts from traditional healing aimed at improving the harmony between mind and body. Approaches in this category include awareness training, breathing techniques and mental imagery. While some mindfulness and mind-body approaches are based on a particular spiritual belief system, you do not need to believe in God or have a spiritual orientation in order to benefit from these practices. Yoga, Tai-chi, and transcendental meditation are examples.

- **Treatments based on scientifically verified forms of energy** including electricity, magnetic fields, light and sound have beneficial effects at many levels in the body and brain. Examples include full-spectrum bright light exposure, weak electrical current, EEG biofeedback, and specialized forms of sound therapy.

- **Treatments based on subtle forms of energy** that have not been verified by science such as Reiki, qigong, prayer, Healing Touch and Therapeutic Touch may be beneficial at the level of postulated energetic processes that may play a role in maintaining optimal physical and psychological wellness, and for treating some mental health problems.

Most vitamins, minerals and essential fatty acids are examples of natural supplements that can be safely used without the advice or supervision of a physician or other health care provider. However, some natural supplements derived from plants or other natural products cause potentially serious safety problems and it is important to adhere to recommended dosages when using these supplements and avoid taking them with prescription medications that are known to cause unsafe toxic interactions.

When a natural supplement is associated with potentially serious adverse effects or toxicities ***important safety warnings are in bold face, underlined and in italics***. ***Before trying any natural supplement that has potentially serious adverse effects, I strongly encourage you to*** ***consult with a knowledgeable health care provider who can advise you about the safe and appropriate use of that supplement***.

While some people prefer to use a medication or a natural supplement only, others benefit from combining a medication or supplement with a whole-body approach, a mind-body practice, or energy work. The treatment plan you decide to use will depend not only on the evidence supporting its use but also the amount of time you have to try a particular approach, and your level of motivation.

Exercise, dietary changes, light exposure therapy, Tai chi, Healing Touch and other therapies may improve symptoms of MCI and mild or moderate dementia. There are no safety concerns when using such approaches while taking a natural supplement or a medication. However, in some cases it takes a great deal of time, effort and experience to use a mind body or energy therapy properly before you can expect to benefit from it.

Finally, you may have a more rapid response if you consistently try recommended dietary changes, regular exercise, or a mind-body practice while also taking an appropriate supplement or a medication. Such combined are examples of integrative mental health care, as described above.

Alternative treatments of MCI and dementia

This section reviews the evidence for specific natural supplements, whole-body approaches, mind-body and mindfulness practices, and energy therapies used to treat MCI and dementia. The information under each treatment approach is listed in bullets so that you can compare research evidence and safety information for a variety of treatment choices:

- Name of treatment and category

- How the treatment works (where known)

- Dosages (for natural supplements) or frequency or duration of use (for whole body, mind-body or energy approaches)

- Examples of safe and effective treatment combinations

- Comments about adverse effects and warnings pertaining to the treatment or treatment combinations that may result in potentially unsafe interactions and should be avoided

- Average duration of treatment needed to achieve beneficial results

I use a 3-tier approach to rate treatments based on the relative strength of evidence.

- **Tier A:** treatments are supported by strong research evidence from rigorously conducted studies or systematic reviews of studies.

- **Tier B:** treatments are also supported by research evidence but not to the same degree as tier A treatments.

- **Tier C:** treatments are supported by weak or inconsistent research findings and may be effective in some cases

Note that treatments under each tier are listed in alphabetical order and not according to the relative strength of evidence.

Tier A treatments of mild cognitive impairment (MCI) and dementia

Dietary changes

Exercise

Ginkgo (*Ginkgo biloba*)

Idebenone

Dietary changes

- **Name of treatment and category:** Dietary factors that reduce the risk of developing dementia include low total fat and caloric intake, high fish consumption, and moderate alcohol consumption. Individuals who drink approximately one glass of wine or beer daily are at significantly less risk of developing dementia compared to non-drinkers or individuals who drink to excess. Long-term adherence to a Mediterranean diet rich in fresh vegetables, fish and olive oil, may be especially beneficial in reducing the risk of developing cognitive decline or dementia. (See also Bredesen protocol which incorporates dietary changes)

- **How the treatment works:** Diets high in fat and total calories promote increased formation of free radicals that damage the brain and increase the risk of dementia and other chronic neurologic and psychiatric disorders. Omega3 fatty acids in some plants and fishes have important anti-inflammatory and neuroprotective effects.

- **Dosages (for natural supplements) or frequency of use (for whole body, mind-body or energy approaches):** There is no professional consensus on causal relationships between specific foods and reduced risk of mild cognitive impairment or dementia.

- **Examples of safe and effective treatment combinations:** Dietary changes are safe in combination with other approaches.

- **Comments about adverse effects and warnings pertaining to treatment combinations that may result in potentially unsafe interactions and should be avoided:** none

- **Average duration of treatment needed to achieve beneficial results:** Long-term adherence to a Mediterranean diet and other specific dietary changes (above) over several years probably reduces the risk of developing dementia or cognitive decline.

Exercise

- **Name of treatment and category:** Exercise is a whole-body approach.

- **How the treatment works:** Regular exercise increases levels of certain factors in the brain that promote new synapse formation and may increase the size of brain regions involved in learning and memory. Regular exercise reduces the risk of dementia in healthy individuals but does *not* lessen the severity of dementia once it has developed.

- **Dosages (for natural supplements) or frequency of use (for whole body, mind-body or energy approaches):** Walking between ¼ mile and 2 miles/daily significantly reduces the risk of developing dementia in healthy elderly individuals.

- **Examples of safe and effective treatment combinations:** Regular exercise may be safely combined with other approaches.

- **Comments about adverse effects and warnings pertaining to treatment combinations that may result in potentially unsafe interactions and should be avoided:** If you have a heart condition, chronic pain or another serious medical condition it is advisable to consult with a physician or other qualified health care provider before starting a regular exercise program.

- **Average duration of treatment needed to achieve beneficial results:** Beneficial effects of on cognitive performance are gradually achieved over several years of regular exercise.

Ginkgo (*Ginkgo biloba*)

- **Name of treatment and category:** Ginkgo (*Ginkgo biloba*) is an herbal widely used in Chinese medicine and other Asian systems of medicine.

- **How the treatment works:** The active ingredients of *G. biloba* have strong anti-oxidant, anti-inflammatory and neuroprotective effects on the brain. A standardized extract of *G. biloba* (EGb 761) may be as effective as some prescription medications for the treatment of moderate but *not* severe symptoms of dementia. *G. biloba* may be most effective in demented individuals who have symptoms of anxiety, depressed mood or apathy.

- **Dosages (for natural supplements) or frequency of use (for whole body, mind-body or energy approaches):** A standardized extract of *G. biloba* (EGb 761) dosed at 120 to

600mg/day in two separate doses reduces the severity of moderate symptoms of dementia in individuals diagnosed with Alzheimer's disease or vascular dementia.

- **Examples of safe and effective treatment combinations:** *G. biloba* may be safely combined with other Chinese herbal medicines e.g. Dangshen (*Codonopsis pilosula*) and Ginseng (*Panax ginseng*), resulting in generally enhanced cognitive functioning. Combining *G. biloba* 240mg/day with a prescription medication used to treat dementia (e.g. donepezil 10mg/day) may be more effective than either treatment alone while reducing adverse effects caused by medication.

- **Comments about adverse effects and warnings pertaining to treatment combinations that may result in potentially unsafe interactions and should be avoided:** *G. biloba* is generally safe when a quality brand is taken at recommended dosages. Some individuals report mild upset stomach, headache or dizziness. ***Caution: G. biloba increases bleeding time and should be discontinued at least 2 weeks before surgery. Warning: G. biloba should not be taken in combination with aspirin, warfarin or other drugs or natural products that interfere with normal bleeding.***

- **Average duration of treatment needed to achieve beneficial results:** A decrease in the severity of dementia may take place after weeks or months of daily treatment with an appropriate dosage of a standardized *G. biloba* preparation.

Idebenone

- **Name of treatment and category:** Idebenone is a semi-synthetic substance that is closely related to coenzyme Q10 (i.e. ubiquinone), a molecule that plays a central role in the body's energy production.

- **How the treatment works:** Idebenone may be a more potent anti-oxidant than coenzyme Q10. It works by increasing energy production in mitochondria inside all cells.

- **Dosages (for natural supplements) or frequency of use (for whole body, mind-body or energy approaches):** Idebenone dosed between 120 and 360mg/day decreases the severity of symptoms of both Alzheimer's dementia and vascular dementia. Some research findings suggest that idebenone may be more effective than prescription medications used to treat dementia.

- **Examples of safe and effective treatment combinations:** There is very little information on combination treatment strategies using idebenone to treat dementia.

- **Comments about adverse effects and warnings pertaining to treatment combinations that may result in potentially unsafe interactions and should be avoided:** none

- **Average duration of treatment needed to achieve beneficial results:** Some individuals diagnosed with dementia experience significant improvement in memory and cognitive functioning after taking idebenone 120mg/day for 3 to 6 months.

Tier B treatments of mild cognitive impairment and dementia

Acetyl-L-carnitine (ALC)

B vitamins (folate, B-12 and thiamin)

Ginseng (*Panax ginseng*)

Herbal formulas: Chotosan (CTS) and Yokukansan (YKS)

Huperzine-A (*Huperzia serrata*)

SLT a Chinese herbal formula

Acetyl-L-carnitine (ALC)

- **Name of treatment and category:** Acetyl-L-carnitine (ALC) occurs naturally in the brain and body and is used as a biological treatment of different medical and mental health problems.

- **How the treatment works:** ALC has general neuroprotective and energy enhancing effects on the brain and may slow the rate of progression of cognitive impairment in normal aging and delay onset of early stages of dementia. ALC may be more effective for symptoms of Alzheimer's dementia than vascular dementia.

- **Dosages (for natural supplements) or frequency of use (for whole body, mind-body or energy approaches):** ALC taken at dosages between 1500 and 3000mg/day may improve memory and general cognitive performance in some individuals diagnosed with mild cognitive impairment or dementia.

- **Examples of safe and effective treatment combinations:** The neuroprotective benefits of ALC may be enhanced when the supplement is taken in combination with coenzyme Q10 or omega3 fatty acids. Preliminary findings suggest that taking a daily formula that includes ALC 500mg, folate 400mg, SAMe 400mg, N-acetyl-cysteine (NAC) 600mg, vitamin B12 6mg, and vitamin E 30 international units (IU), may reduce the rate of progression of cognitive decline in individuals diagnosed with early Alzheimer's dementia, improve symptoms of depressed mood and reduce disruptive behavior.

- **Comments about adverse effects and warnings pertaining to treatment combinations that may result in potentially unsafe interactions and should be avoided:** ALC is generally well tolerated and may be safely combined with other natural products (above) and prescription medications. Some individuals experience nausea, diarrhea, headache or upset stomach. There are uncommon reports of elevated blood pressure and increased heart rate.

- **Average duration of treatment needed to achieve beneficial results:** Some Individuals with mild or moderate dementia experience improvements in memory, cognition and depressed mood after taking the above dosage of ALC or a multi-nutrient formula that includes ALC for several months.

B vitamins (folate, B-12 and thiamin)

- **Name of treatment and category:** folate (also called folic acid, methylfolinic acid and l-methylfolate), B-12 (cobalamin) and thiamin are naturally occurring members of the B vitamin family found in many foods and are widely used to treat different medical and mental health problems and improve overall health.

- **How the treatment works:** Certain B vitamins are necessary for making brain chemicals that are essential for memory and normal cognitive functioning. Chronic inadequate folate and B-12 in the diet results in impaired cognition and memory.

- **Dosages or frequency of use (for whole body, mind-body or energy approaches):** Dietary folate below 400 micrograms/day is associated with an increased risk of becoming demented. Folate in the form of methyl-folinic acid 50mg/day may decrease symptoms of dementia and depressed mood in persons in the early stages of Alzheimer's disease. B-12 may be taken as a subcutaneous injection, as a nasal spray or a tablet placed beneath the tongue. B-12 dosed at 1mg/week may reduce the rate of normal age-related cognitive decline in the elderly and provide beneficial cognitive enhancing effects in moderately demented individuals. Thiamin dosed at 3 to 8gm/day may decrease the severity of mild to moderate dementia.

- **Examples of safe and effective treatment combinations:** Many individuals take a daily B-complex that contains all B vitamins at recommended daily dosages for maintaining good health. B vitamins may be safely combined with other treatment approaches.

- **Comments about adverse effects and warnings pertaining to treatment combinations that may result in potentially unsafe interactions and should be avoided:** High doses of folate (above 15mg/day) may cause nervousness, restlessness, insomnia or agitation. *<u>Caution: taking a high dose folate supplement in the absence of folate deficiency may cause harmful effects and may mask B-12 deficiency. It is prudent to check the blood folate level to find out if the level is abnormally low before considering taking a high dose folate supplement.</u>*

- **Average duration of treatment needed to achieve beneficial results:** Vitamin B supplementation may be safely continued on a long-term basis. Some individuals experience moderate improvements in memory and general cognitive functioning after taking one or more of the above B vitamins for weeks or longer.

Ginseng (*Panax ginseng*)

Name of treatment and category: *P. ginseng* (also known as Asian ginseng or Korean ginseng) is a widely used herbal in Asia and the West to treat medical and mental health problems.

- **How the treatment works:** Ginseng belongs to a family of herbals called *adaptogens* because it improves stamina and feelings of general wellbeing and enhances the body's capacity to deal with chronic stress. Ginseng contains biomolecules that have anti-inflammatory and antioxidant properties which contribute to beneficial effects on memory and cognition. There is evidence that an active ingredient of ginseng may inhibit the enzyme that breaks down acetylcholine between synapses, resulting in increased brain levels of a neurotransmitter that plays an important role in memory and cognition. This is the mechanism underlying widely prescribed medications for Alzheimer's disease, the cholinesterase inhibitors.

- **Dosages (for natural supplements) or frequency of use (for whole body, mind-body or energy approaches):** In a small placebo-controlled study, individuals with Alzheimer's disease treated with a high dose (9gm/day) or low dose (4.5gm/day) of standardized extract of *P. ginseng* experienced significant improvements in memory and cognitive function compared to those receiving a placebo.
- **Examples of safe and effective treatment combinations: One small study showed that a standardized extract of P. ginseng can be a beneficial add-on therapy to conventional treatment with cholinesterase inhibitor possibly increasing effectiveness. The combination was well tolerated.**

- **Comments about adverse effects and warnings pertaining to treatment combinations that may result in potentially unsafe interactions and should be avoided:** Ginseng preparations are generally well tolerated when taken at recommended dosages. Uncommon side effects include headaches, upset stomach and insomnia. Ginseng interacts with some medications including anticoagulant agents, some antidepressants (especially monoamine oxidase inhibitors) and the mood stabilizer lamotrigine potentially resulting in toxicity. These combinations should be avoided.
- **Average duration of treatment needed to achieve beneficial results:** Some individuals with early or moderate Alzheimer's disease experience significant and sustained improvements in short-term memory and cognition after taking a standardized extract of *P. ginseng* at the above dosages for 12 weeks. In a long-term study, individuals who received 4.5 or 9gm/day of a standardized *P. ginseng* extract remained at their previous cognitive baseline after 2

years. Maximum improvement in cognitive functioning was observed after 24 weeks of treatment.

Herbal formulas: Chotosan (CTS) and Yokukansan (YKS)

- **Name of treatment and category:** The same two herbal formulas are used in both traditional Japanese Kampo medicine and Traditional Chinese medicine to treat symptoms of dementia and cognitive decline. In Kampo they are called *Chotosan* (CTS) and *Yokukansan* (YKS). In Chinese medicine the same two herbal formulas are called *Gouteng-san* and *Yigan-san*. CTS contains 11 distinct herbals whereas YKS contains 7 herbal ingredients. Both formulas contain *Uncariae Uncis cum Ramulus* which is believed to play an important role in decreasing the severity of cognitive symptoms.

- **How the treatment works:** Both formulas have potent antioxidant activity, increase the levels of neurotransmitters involved in learning and memory, and may enhance neural plasticity. CTS and YKS improve global cognitive functioning, enhance activities of daily living, and decrease the severity of confusion, hallucinations, agitation and disturbed sleep in demented individuals. Research findings suggest YKS may be beneficial for many kinds of dementia including dementia related to Parkinson's disease, fronto-temporal dementia, Lewy body dementia, vascular dementia and Alzheimer's disease. In Japan YKS is widely prescribed for depressed mood and anxiety conditions, problems that often accompany cognitive decline and dementia.

- **Dosages or frequency of use (for whole body, mind-body or energy approaches):** For both CTS and YKS an extract prepared from 7.5g of the dry herbal formula is taken daily.

- **Examples of safe and effective treatment combinations:** Both herbal preparations may be safely combined with prescription medications used to treat dementia. Some individuals who take CTS or YKS are able to decrease their usual daily dosage of antipsychotic medications (i.e. used to treat behavioral symptoms of dementia) without symptomatic worsening.

- **Comments about adverse effects and warnings pertaining to treatment combinations that may result in potentially unsafe interactions and should be avoided:** CTS and YKS are generally safe with few reports of mild adverse effects when taken alone or in combination with prescription medications.

- **Average duration of treatment needed to achieve beneficial results:** Studies done on both herbal formulas showed significant improvement in symptoms of dementia after 4 weeks of daily treatment at the above dosages.

Huperzine-A (*Huperzia serrata*)

- **Name of treatment and category:** Huperzine-A is derived from the herb *H. serrata*, and is a component of many Chinese herbal formulas used to treat cognitive problems.

- **How the treatment works:** Huperzine-A has beneficial neuroprotective effects on the brain.

- **Dosages or frequency of use (for whole body, mind-body or energy approaches):** A standardized extract of Huperzine-A dosed between 200 and 400 micrograms/day has general beneficial effects delaying the rate of progression of Alzheimer's dementia and vascular dementia and slowing the rate of normal age-related cognitive decline.

- **Examples of safe and effective treatment combinations:** Additive beneficial effects on cognitive functioning may occur when Huperzine A is used in combination with green tea.

- **Comments about adverse effects and warnings pertaining to treatment combinations that may result in potentially unsafe interactions and should be avoided:** Some individuals who take huperzine-A experience dry mouth, diarrhea, nausea or mild dizziness. *<u>Caution: Huperzine-A should be avoided during pregnancy and in nursing mothers.</u>*

- **Average duration of treatment needed to achieve beneficial results:** Persons diagnosed with dementia may experience significant improvements in cognitive functioning and their capacity to perform activities of daily living after taking Huperzine-A at the above dosage for several weeks.

SLT (a compound herbal formula)

- **Name of treatment and category:** SLT is a compound herbal formula that consists of *Ginkgo biloba* (ginkgo),

Panax ginseng (ginseng), and *Crocus sativus* (saffron) extracts.

- **How the treatment works:** The formula is believed to improve memory and cognition through the combined antioxidant and neuroprotective mechanisms of all three herbals (see separate entries). Animal studies have established that SLT decreases areas of focal cerebral ischemia following stroke, decreased platelet aggregation, and increase free radical scavenging activity, all of which may contribute to improved memory and cognitive function. Human studies have shown that SLT improves memory and cognition in healthy adults and mitigates symptoms of memory loss and cognitive impairment in individuals with mild to moderate symptoms of vascular dementia. **NOTE: at the time of writing (October 2019) available pharmacologic and other mainstream medical treatments are *ineffective* against vascular dementia. In the past few years large multi-center placebo-controlled**

human clinical trials have consistently reported significant beneficial effects of SLT on memory loss and other symptoms of vascular dementia. Pending confirmation by a phase III multi-center clinical trial SLT may prove to be one of the most important breakthroughs in the treatment of vascular dementia.

- **Dosages (for natural supplements) or frequency of use (for whole body, mind-body or energy approaches):** Findings of large multi-center human clinical trials show that a standardized formula of SLT dosed at 240 to 360mg/day improves memory and general cognitive functioning in individuals with mild to moderate vascular dementia.
- **Examples of safe and effective treatment combinations:** *G. biloba,* a component of SLT, may be safely combined with cholinesterase inhibitors possibly increasing efficacy and reducing adverse effects.
- **Comments about adverse effects and warnings pertaining to treatment combinations that may result in potentially**

unsafe interactions and should be avoided: Large multi-center studies on SLT in vascular dementia have reported no serious adverse effects. However, the safety considerations for Ginkgo biloba (ginkgo), Panax ginseng (ginseng), and Crocus sativus (saffron) when taken separately should be kept in mind when considering using the SLT formula in combination with any medication. Further, there may be potential safety concerns when combining SLT with another natural product or psychotropic medication that have not yet been identified through animal or human trials. For example, G. biloba interferes with normal blood clotting and should be avoided before surgery or in individuals taking blood thinners. *Caution: until there is reliable safety information on combined regimens of SLT and dementia medications from animal studies or human clinical trials, it is prudent to avoid combining SLT with medications used to treat dementia.*

- **Average duration of treatment needed to achieve beneficial results:** Healthy adults report improved cognitive functioning after taking SLT at the above dosages for 1 week. Individuals with mild to moderate vascular dementia experience significant improvements in memory and cognition after 6 months to one year of daily SLT.

Tier C treatments of mild cognitive impairment and dementia

Bright light exposure therapy

Cranial electrical stimulation (CES) and transcutaneous electrical stimulation (TENS)

Curcumin (*Curcuma longa*)

Healing Touch (HT) and Therapeutic Touch (TT)

Lavender (*Lavandula angustifolia*) and lemon balm (*Melissa officinalis*)

Massage

Melatonin

Multi-modality protocols

Music

Nicotinamide adenine dinucleotide (NAD+)

Qigong and Tai Chi

Resveratrol

Saffron (Crocus sativus)

Snoezelen

Transcranial photobiomodulation

Vitamins C (ascorbic acid) and E (alpha tocopherol)

Wander gardens

Bright light exposure therapy

- **Name of treatment and category:** bright light exposure is a scientifically validated energy therapy.

- **How the treatment works:** Timed exposure to bright full spectrum light using a light box, light visor or ceiling lights may influence the body's *biological clocks* (which may not be functioning normally in individuals diagnosed with dementia) resulting in improved sleep, enhanced mood, decreased symptoms of restlessness and agitation, and increased capacity to perform daily activities.

- **Dosages (for natural supplements) or frequency of use (for whole body, mind-body or energy approaches):** Studies on the effects of bright light on behavior in individuals diagnosed with dementia have investigated brief exposure to bright full spectrum light (ranging in intensity from 2,500 to 10,000 lux) at different times of day, and all-day exposure to full-spectrum ceiling lights (approximately 1000 lux).

- **Examples of safe and effective treatment combinations:** bright light exposure therapy may be safely used in combination with other approaches.

- **Comments about adverse effects and warnings pertaining to treatment combinations that may result in potentially unsafe interactions and should be avoided:** none

- **Average duration of treatment needed to achieve beneficial results:** Some demented individuals experience moderate improvement in sleep and depressed mood after several weeks of daily bright light therapy.

Cranial electrical stimulation (CES) and transcutaneous electrical stimulation (TENS)

- **Name of treatment and category:** CES and TENS are scientifically validated energy therapies in which electrodes are used to deliver a very weak electrical current into the head, neck or back.

- **How the treatment works:** Regular electrical stimulation of the brain may have beneficial effects on brain chemistry resulting in improvements in memory and general cognitive functioning. Some individuals diagnosed with dementia experience transient improvements in disturbed sleep, word recall and facial recognition immediately following treatment.

- **Dosages (for natural supplements) or frequency of use (for whole body, mind-body or energy approaches):** A pulsed electrical current with a specialized *shape* at a frequency between 0.5 and 2 Hz (i.e. cycles per second) and a power of 10 to 100 micro-Amps is applied at two electrodes attached to the mid-back (TENS) or the earlobes (CES). Sessions usually last 30 minutes and are self-administered 5 days per week for several weeks.

- **Examples of safe and effective treatment combinations:** CES and TENS may be safely used in combination with other approaches.

- **Comments about adverse effects and warnings pertaining to treatment combinations that may result in potentially unsafe interactions and should be avoided:** CES and TENS are generally safe when recommended guidelines are followed. Some individuals experience mild tingling sensations. *<u>Caution: CES may cause an abnormal heart rhythm and should not be used by anyone who has a cardiac pacemaker.</u>*

- **Average duration of treatment needed to achieve beneficial results:** some individuals experience improvements in word recall, facial recognition and motivation following several CES or TENS treatments when pulsed electrical current is applied to the head or back.

Curcumin (*Curcuma longa*)

- **Name of treatment and category:** Curcumin, derived from the root of turmeric (*Curcuma longa*), is an important herbal used in Indian cooking and Ayurvedic medicine.

- **How the treatment works:** Curcumin has potent neuroprotective and anti-oxidant effects. Findings of studies on curcumin for dementia are highly inconsistent and vary with respect to study design, dosage and other factors. However, some individuals diagnosed with Alzheimer's disease experience moderate improvement in cognition and memory, and reductions in symptoms of agitation, irritability and apathy that frequently accompany dementia.

- **Dosages (for natural supplements) or frequency of use (for whole body, mind-body or energy approaches):** The optimal dosage of curcumin for the treatment of dementia has not been established. For purposes of treating Alzheimer's disease, a dry curcumin preparation is often taken at a dosage ranging from 100mg to 4gm/day. **NOTE: Most currently available curcumin preparations are poorly absorbed through the gut. Ongoing research efforts to develop curcumin preparations that are more readily absorbed may enhance the effectiveness the herbal as a treatment of dementia.**

- **Examples of safe and effective treatment combinations:** Curcumin may be safely combined with other natural supplements and prescription medications. Some individuals diagnosed with Alzheimer's disease benefit from a combined regimen of curcumin and *G. biloba*.

- **Comments about adverse effects and warnings pertaining to treatment combinations that may result in potentially unsafe interactions and should be avoided:** Curcumin is generally safe. Some individuals experience mild adverse effects including headache, diarrhea and skin rash.

- **Average duration of treatment needed to achieve beneficial results:** Some individuals experience decreased severity of dementia after taking a quality preparation of curcumin for several months.

Healing touch (HT) and Therapeutic touch (TT)

- **Name of treatment and category:** Healing Touch (HT) and Therapeutic Touch (TT) are energetic therapies that have not been scientifically validated.

- **How the treatment works:** Limited research findings suggest that HT and TT may decrease agitation and disruptive behavior in individuals diagnosed with Alzheimer's disease or other forms of dementia.

- **Dosages (for natural supplements) or frequency of use (for whole body, mind-body or energy approaches):** HT and TT treatments are administered by certified practitioners in brief 10 to 20-minute sessions daily or more often depending on the severity of agitation or disruptive behavior.

- **Examples of safe and effective treatment combinations:** HT and TT may be safely combined with other approaches.

- **Comments about adverse effects and warnings pertaining to treatment combinations that may result in potentially unsafe interactions and should be avoided:** none

- **Average duration of treatment needed to achieve beneficial results:** Some demented individuals experience decreases in agitation after days or weeks of regular HT or TT therapy.

Lavender (*Lavandula angustifolia*) and lemon balm (*Melissa officinalis*)

- **Name of treatment and category:** Essential oils of lavender (*Lavandula angustifolia*) and lemon balm (*Melissa* *officinalis*) can be inhaled as aromatherapy or applied directly to the skin.

- **How the treatment works:** The essential oils of lavender and lemon balm may have beneficial calming effects on agitation in demented persons however research findings are limited and inconsistent. The essential oils of both herbals reduce the levels of stress hormones in the blood and have beneficial effects on several neurotransmitters resulting in general feelings of calmness. Essential oils are probably absorbed better and are more effective when applied to the skin. ***Aromatherapy is probably not an effective treatment of agitation in demented individuals***.

- **Dosages (for natural supplements) or frequency of use (for whole body, mind-body or energy approaches):** There is no agreement on standardized dosages of essential oils for the treatment of agitation or disruptive behavior in dementia however some researchers have reported temporary decreases in agitation when 1ml of a concentrated preparation of lavender oil or lemon balm (30%) is applied to the forearms and face. Many demented individuals experience significant reductions in agitated behavior and improved quality of life when the above essential oils are applied twice daily.

- **Examples of safe and effective treatment combinations:** Most essential oils are safe when used in combination with other approaches.

- **Comments about adverse effects and warnings pertaining to treatment combinations that may result in potentially unsafe interactions and should be avoided:** Essential oils are generally safe when used appropriately at the above dosages. Uncommon minor adverse effects include allergic skin reactions and a photosensitive rash. The essential oils of lavender and lemon balm may increase the sedating effects of prescription tranquilizers. ***Caution: pregnant*** *women should not apply essential oils to the skin to avoid possible toxicity to the fetus.*

- **Average duration of treatment needed to achieve beneficial results:** some individuals diagnosed with dementia experience reductions in agitated behavior after 2 to 4 weeks of regular daily use of the above essential oils.

Massage therapy

- **Name of treatment and category:** massage is a whole-body approach.

- **How the treatment works:** Gentle massage produces general calming effects. Limited research findings suggest that light pressure massage may reduce the severity of agitation and inappropriate behavior in individuals diagnosed with dementia.

- **Dosages (for natural supplements) or frequency of use (for whole body, mind-body or energy approaches):** Light massage for 10 to 15 minutes applied to the head, shoulders and hands may be especially effective in reducing agitation and inappropriate behavior in demented persons. Massage is probably most effective at reducing agitation if provided at times when agitation or inappropriate behaviors are more likely to occur.

- **Examples of safe and effective treatment combinations:** Massage may be safely combined with other approaches.

- **Comments about adverse effects and warnings pertaining to treatment combinations that may result in potentially unsafe interactions and should be avoided:** none

- **Average duration of treatment needed to achieve beneficial results:** The calming effects of gentle massage in persons diagnosed with dementia take place immediately and last for a short time afterwards.

Melatonin

- **Name of treatment and category:** Melatonin is a hormone that occurs naturally in the brain and is used as a biological treatment.

- **How the treatment works:** Melatonin regulates the sleep-wake cycle and has strong neuroprotective effects.

- **Dosages (for natural supplements) or frequency of use (for whole body, mind-body or energy approaches):** Taking 3 to 24mg of a fast release preparation of melatonin 30 minutes before bedtime may reduce agitated behavior in individuals diagnosed with dementia and slow the overall rate of cognitive decline in both dementia and mild cognitive impairment.

- **Examples of safe and effective treatment combinations:** Melatonin may be safely used in combination with other natural supplements and prescription medications. Taking melatonin with a sedative-hypnotic may permit reduction of the dose needed to sleep.

- **Comments about adverse effects and warnings pertaining to treatment combinations that may result in potentially unsafe interactions and should be avoided:** Melatonin is generally safe, has few minor adverse effects and is mildly sedating even when taken at high doses.

- **Average duration of treatment needed to achieve beneficial results:** Some individuals diagnosed with dementia or mild cognitive impairment experience improvements in sleep and cognition after several weeks of nightly melatonin use. Melatonin should be taken on an on-going basis for consistent beneficial effects on cognitive functioning.

Multi-modality protocols

- **Name of treatment and category:** Multi-modality treatment protocols such as the Bredesen protocol are personalized comprehensive lifestyle and nutrition programs.

- **How the treatment works: (NOTE: compare different approaches if there are data)** The Bredesen Protocol targets 36 biochemical and metabolic factors that contribute to development of Alzheimer's disease and prescribes an individualized treatment plan of diet, supplements, sleep, exercise and other lifestyle modifications with the goal of reversing the causes of Alzheimer's disease. Beneficial effects achieved through dietary modification, regular exercise, stress management or a mindfulness practice, and supplementation with natural products may involve different mechanisms of action at multiple levels in the body and brain including enhanced immune function; reduced insulin resistance; reduced inflammation; reduced brain atrophy and stimulation of new synapse formation. It is important to note that all findings to date are based on a small number of dramatic case reports. Although these findings are promising they should be viewed as preliminary pending completion of a large clinical trial that is on-going at the time of writing (October, 2019).

- **Dosages (for natural supplements) or frequency of use (for whole body, mind-body or energy approaches):** Patients who follow the Bredesen protocol are encouraged to strictly adhere to all recommended lifestyle changes, nutrition advice and supplementation with select natural products. The protocol includes the following specific recommendations:

  - Adherence to a low-glycemic diet
  - 12-hour fast each night (including 3 hours before bedtime)
  - consumption of probiotic-rich foods like plain Greek yogurt, kombucha, kefir, and fermented foods like miso and sauerkraut, and antioxidant-rich foods like blueberries and blackberries

- 8 hours sleep every night, treating sleep apnea when it is present and use of melatonin if needed
- a regular mind-body or mindfulness practice
- regular exercise 30 to 60 minutes 4 to six times a week
- Vitamin B-12 (goal is serum vitamin B-12 levels higher than 500)
- Curcumin 400 to 500mg 3 to 4 times daily (taken with meals for better absorption) (please see separate entry on Curcumin)
- citicoline 1000 to 2000mg and the omega-3 fatty acid (DHA) (see separate entry on omega-3s)
- daily supplementation with vitamin D3 in individuals with vitamin D deficiency vitamin E 400 mg (mixed tocopherols and tocotrienols); vitamin C 500-1,000 mg
- alpha lipoic acid 200 mg

- **Examples of safe and effective treatment combinations:** The Bredesen protocol can be followed in combination with other approaches.

- **Comments about adverse effects and warnings pertaining to treatment combinations that may result in potentially unsafe interactions and should be avoided:** none

- **Average duration of treatment needed to achieve beneficial results:** In a case series 9 out of 10 individuals with MCI or early Alzheimer's disease experienced significant improvement in memory and other areas of cognitive functioning after closely following the protocol for 3 to 6 months.

Music

- **Name of treatment and category:** Music is a scientifically validated energy therapy.

- **How the treatment works:** Listening to music, singing and playing games that involve music may decrease agitation and improve mood and cognitive functioning in individuals diagnosed with dementia. Music therapy is an important part of a comprehensive care plan for demented individuals who live in residential care settings.

- **Dosages (for natural supplements) or frequency of use (for whole body, mind-body or energy approaches):** There is no consensus on the *optimal* amount of listening time needed to achieve calming effects. Some residential care programs provide music therapy twice weekly or more often.

- **Examples of safe and effective treatment combinations:** Music therapy may be safely used in combination with all other approaches.

- **Comments about adverse effects and warnings pertaining to treatment combinations that may result in potentially unsafe interactions and should be avoided:** none

- **Average duration of treatment needed to achieve beneficial results:** Some individuals diagnosed with dementia may experience moderate reductions in agitation after several weeks of regular music therapy. One small study found that twice daily exposure to calming music *slightly improved* cognitive functioning after one year.

Nicotinamide adenine dinucleotide (NAD+)

- **Name of treatment and category:** NAD+ is a naturally occurring molecule in mitochondria, the 'power houses' of all cells.
- **How the treatment works:** NAD+ is essential for normal mitochondrial function and is required for neuronal energy production needed for memory and cognitive function. NAD+ is an essential co-factor for DNA repair and cellular metabolism. NAD+ levels decline with normal aging resulting in age-related memory problems. High rates of NAD+ depletion caused by oxidative stress in the brain may contribute to neuropathological changes that eventually result in Alzheimer's disease and other degenerative neurologic diseases. Findings of animal studies suggest that supplementation with NAD+ precursors like nicotinamide riboside (NR), nicotinamide mononucleotide (NMN), and nicotinamide (NAM) lessens DNA damage, improves general health, prolongs longevity. Beneficial effects of NAD+ precursors on the brain include decreasing synaptic

dysfunction and slowing down of the rate of neuronal degeneration, possibly mitigating the progressive neuropathological changes that eventually lead to AD and other neurodegenerative diseases.

- **Dosages (for natural supplements) or frequency of use (for whole body, mind-body or energy approaches):** Optimal dosages of NAD+ precursors in humans have not been determined. In one study healthy individuals taking NR 1000 mg/day had a 2.7-fold increase in NAD+ levels and a 45-fold increase in NR levels. In a small 6-month study individuals with AD taking NAD+ 10mg/day continued to function at their cognitive baseline with no declines in reasoning and memory.
- **Examples of safe and effective treatment combinations:** unknown.
- **Comments about adverse effects and warnings pertaining to treatment combinations that may result in potentially unsafe interactions and should be avoided:** There have

been no reports of serious adverse effects in animals when NAD+ precursors are taken at dosages up to 1000mg/kg. Studies assessing safety of NAD+ precursors are ongoing.

- **Average duration of treatment needed to achieve beneficial results:** There is insufficient data to determine whether there is an optimal duration of treatment with NAD+ to result in beneficial effects on MCI or AD.

Qigong and Tai Chi

- **Name of treatment and category:** Qigong and Tai Chi are mind-body practices that combine movement and meditation. While Tai Chi involves elaborate dance-like sequences of movements, Qigong exercises consist of simple repetitive movements. Both approaches are used for maintaining wellness and treating different medical and mental health problems.

- **How the treatment works:** The regular practice of qigong or Tai Chi has beneficial calming effects. In Chinese medical theory both approaches are regarded as *energetic* practices that restore the body and mind to optimal balance. The regular practice of qigong or Tai Chi improves balance, strength and flexibility. Limited research findings suggest that the regular practice of qigong may decrease the severity of chronic pain disorders, reduce fatigue and enhance immune functioning.

- **Dosages (for natural supplements) or frequency of use (for whole body, mind-body or energy approaches):** Limited findings suggest that the regular practice of simple qigong exercises may reduce agitation in individuals diagnosed with Alzheimer's disease or other kinds of dementia.

- **Examples of safe and effective treatment combinations:** Tai Chi and qigong may be safely used in combination with other approaches.

- **Comments about adverse effects and warnings pertaining to treatment combinations that may result in potentially**

unsafe interactions and should be avoided: Qigong and Tai Chi are generally safe when practiced under the supervision or with the guidance of a skilled teacher. ***Caution: some Qigong exercises are activating, may potentially worsen symptoms of agitation and should thus be avoided in individuals diagnosed with dementia. Instruction in appropriate qigong exercises for individuals diagnosed with dementia should be obtained from a qualified Qigong teacher.***

- **Average duration of treatment needed to achieve beneficial results:** Some individuals diagnosed with dementia experience general calming benefits after several weeks of regular qigong practice.

Resveratrol

- **Name of treatment and category:** Resveratrol is derived from the skins and seeds of red grapes, is naturally present in red wine and is used as a biological treatment.

- **How the treatment works:** Resveratrol has potent anti-inflammatory, anti-oxidant, neuroprotective and anti-cancer effects. Resveratrol interferes with pathological processes in the brain that manifest as Alzheimer's disease. **NOTE: although resveratrol holds promise as a significant future treatment of Alzheimer's disease most research to date has been done on animal models.**

- **Dosages (for natural supplements) or frequency of use (for whole body, mind-body or energy approaches):** An optimal dosage of resveratrol for the treatment of dementia has not been established. Currently available forms of resveratrol are difficult to absorb through the gut resulting in negligible availability in the brain even with large dosages. **NOTE: Research efforts are ongoing to develop more stable forms of resveratrol that are more readily absorbed in the gut and pass into the brain at levels that** may have more consistent beneficial effects on cognitive functioning.

- **Examples of safe and effective treatment combinations:** Resveratrol may be safely combined with most other biological treatments.

- **Comments about adverse effects and warnings pertaining to treatment combinations that may result in potentially unsafe interactions and should be avoided:** Findings of animal studies suggest that resveratrol is non-toxic even when taken at high dosages. *<u>Caution: studies evaluating safety of resveratrol in humans have not been done.</u>*

- **Average duration of treatment needed to achieve beneficial results:** The duration of treatment with resveratrol needed to achieve beneficial effects on cognitive functioning in dementia has not been determined and will probably depend on the severity of cognitive symptoms being treated, absorption in the gut, and bioavailability in the brain of products currently under development.

Saffron (*Crocus sativus*)

- **Name of treatment and category:** Saffron is obtained from the flowers of the herbal *Crocus sativus* and is used as a biological treatment of different medical and mental health problems.

- **How the treatment works:** Saffron has potent anti-oxidant and neuroprotective effects and may inhibit formation of amyloid plaque in the brain, a known cause of Alzheimer's disease. Saffron affects the same neurotransmitters involved in learning and memory that are targeted by currently available prescription medications used to treat Alzheimer's disease. **NOTE: Saffron has established antidepressant effects and is a reasonable choice for individuals diagnosed with dementia who also have depressed mood.**

- **Dosages (for natural supplements) or frequency of use (for whole body, mind-body or energy approaches):** A saffron extract dosed at 30mg/day may be as effective as currently available prescription medications for slowing the rate of cognitive deterioration in individuals with moderate to severe Alzheimer's disease.

- **Examples of safe and effective treatment combinations:** There are no documented toxic interactions between saffron and prescription medications thus saffron can probably be safely used in combination with prescription medications. Saffron may be safely combined with antidepressants and other prescription medications.

- **Comments about adverse effects and warnings pertaining to treatment combinations that may result in potentially unsafe interactions and should be avoided:** None.

- **Average duration of treatment needed to achieve beneficial results:** Some individuals with moderate to severe Alzheimer's disease experience slowing in the rate of progression of cognitive decline when taking 30mg/day of a standardized saffron extract.

Snoezelen

- **Name of treatment and category:** Snoezelen is a whole-body approach based on stimulation of all the senses (i.e. sight, smell, touch, etc) with the goal of enhancing cognitive functioning in individuals diagnosed with dementia.

- **How the treatment works:** An occupational therapist trained in Snoezelen guides the demented individual through several exercises that aim to stimulate different senses. Limited research has been done on Snoezelen for agitated behavior in dementia. Regular Snoezelen therapy may enhance sensory integration, improve general cognitive functioning and decrease symptoms of apathy and agitation in some demented individuals.

- **Dosages (for natural supplements) or frequency of use (for whole body, mind-body or energy approaches):** Many nursing homes offer Snoezelen to demented individuals 2 or 3 times weekly as part of a comprehensive care program.

- **Examples of safe and effective treatment combinations:** Snoezelen therapy may be safely combined with other therapies.

- **Comments about adverse effects and warnings pertaining to treatment combinations that may result in potentially unsafe interactions and should be avoided:** none

- **Average duration of treatment needed to achieve beneficial results:** Some demented individuals experience benefits after 4 to 8 Snoezelen sessions.

Transcranial photobiomodulation

- **Name of treatment and category:** transcranial photobiomodulation, also called transcranial low-level laser therapy (TLLLT), is a scientifically validated energy therapy that is widely used to accelerate wound healing, reduce pain associated with diabetic peripheral neuropathy, and to treat other medical problems.

- **How the treatment works:** TLLLT uses a light-emitting diode (LED) or low-power laser diode to deliver red to near infrared light (at wavelengths between 600 and 1100 nm across the skull with the goal of modulating neuronal activity. The mechanism of action is believed to involve the stimulation of increased ATP production in mitochondria and neuroprotective effects that reduce neuronal cell death in certain brain regions. Early research findings suggest that TLLLT holds promise for delaying or preventing cognitive decline in individuals diagnosed with early Alzheimer's disease and vascular dementia. Researchers feel that TLLLT will probably not benefit individuals beyond the first stages of Alzheimer's disease who already have extensive irreversible brain damage.

- **Dosages (for natural supplements) or frequency of use (for whole body, mind-body or energy approaches):** In small sham-controlled studies both healthy adults and individuals with MCI treated with TLLLT using light in the red or near infra-red range consisting of 8 minutes administered in eight 1-min treatments alternating between two locations on the forehead, exhibited more improvement in a standardized test of executive functioning compared to individuals randomized to sham treatment consisting of lower energy light. These findings are highly preliminary and *the optimal wavelength, duration, dose and power density for TLLLT treatment have not been determined.*

- **Examples of safe and effective treatment combinations:** TLLLT may be safely used with other treatments.

- **Comments about adverse effects and warnings pertaining to treatment combinations that may result in potentially unsafe interactions and should be avoided:** Serious toxic reactions or adverse effects to TLLLT have not been reported.

- **Average duration of treatment needed to achieve beneficial results:** Findings of a small single-blind pilot study in 19 patients with MCI showed significant improvement in memory and global cognitive functioning after 12 weeks of TLLLT. Important unanswered questions include: how long the beneficial effects of TLLLT last, whether repeated TLLLT treatments are necessary, and whether a plateau is reached after which there may be no further benefit.

Vitamins C (ascorbic acid) and E (alpha tocopherol)

- **Name of treatment and category:** Vitamin C and E are naturally occurring vitamins used to treat different medical and mental health problems.

- **How the treatment works:** Vitamins C and E are potent anti-oxidants that play important neuroprotective roles in the brain. High doses of vitamin C may reduce pathological changes in the brain (i.e. the formation of amyloid plaque) that eventually lead to Alzheimer's disease. Vitamin C is essential for the synthesis of neurotransmitters required for normal cognitive functioning such as serotonin and dopamine.

- **Dosages (for natural supplements) or frequency of use (for whole body, mind-body or energy approaches):** A combined daily regimen of vitamin C (at least 500mg/day) and vitamin E (at least 400 IU/day) may reduce the risk of developing Alzheimer's disease and slow the rate of progression of dementia. <u>*NOTE: Taking vitamin C or E alone probably does not decrease the risk of dementia.*</u>

- **Examples of safe and effective treatment combinations:** Vitamin C and E may be safely combined with other natural products or prescription medications.

- **Comments about adverse effects and warnings pertaining to treatment combinations that may result in potentially unsafe interactions and should be avoided:** *Caution: high doses of vitamin E increase the risk of bleeding. Caution: vitamin E should not be taken by individuals who are at risk of stroke or who take aspirin or another blood thinner.*

- **Average duration of treatment needed to achieve beneficial results:** Some demented individuals experience moderate improvements in cognition after several months on a daily regimen that includes vitamin C and E.

Wander gardens (also called therapeutic gardens, sensory gardens or healing gardens)

- **Name of treatment and category:** A *wander garden* is an outdoor area intended for use by individuals diagnosed with dementia or other severe neuropsychological disorders. Wander gardens provide safe environments where cognitively impaired individuals can walk, socialize and explore nature.

- **How the treatment works:** Wander gardens provide stimulation to all the senses while providing a pleasurable experience and a sense of self-sufficiency to individuals diagnosed with dementia. Regular access to a wander garden may increase positive social contact, improve mood, reduce inappropriate behaviors, improve general quality of life, reduce the use of psychotropic medications (including antipsychotics used to treat aggressive or disruptive behavior) and associated adverse effects, and reduce fall risk.

- **Dosages (for natural supplements) or frequency of use (for whole body, mind-body or energy approaches):** Many residential facilities have programs that allow residents access to a wander garden 3 times weekly or more often for 45 minutes at a time.

- **Examples of safe and effective treatment combinations:** Access to wander gardens may be safely combined with all other approaches.

- **Comments about adverse effects and warnings pertaining to treatment combinations that may result in potentially unsafe interactions and should be avoided:** none

- **Average duration of treatment needed to achieve beneficial results:** Some individuals diagnosed with dementia experience symptomatic improvement after several weeks of regular access to a wander garden.

Before starting treatment

The treatment or treatment combinations you decide to try after reading this book will be based on your unique history, symptoms, preferences and circumstances. As you learn how to think about your mental health care in a more holistic way using the concepts and information in this book you will discover a variety of ways to manage symptoms of mild cognitive impairment or dementia.

Before starting one or more treatments I encourage you to finish reading the entire book to make sure you know how to develop a plan that is *appropriate for you or a person you are caring for*. If in addition to MCI or dementia, you or someone you are caring for have another mental health problem, I encourage you to read the book in the series on that condition or find another reliable source of information before starting any new treatment.

Developing a treatment plan that is *appropriate for you or a person you are caring for*

General considerations

Now that you've learned about a variety of alternative treatment choices the next step is to decide on treatments that address your particular symptoms keeping in mind treatment choices that are available where you live and within your budget.

As I mentioned earlier, because everyone's psychological and medical history and symptoms are unique the best treatment plan for you or a person you are caring for may be very different from the most appropriate treatment for someone else. In other words, **there is no single best treatment for everyone with MCI or dementia.**

The best treatment plan *for you or a person you are caring for* is based on:

- research evidence
- response to previously tried treatments

- personal preferences
- treatments that are available where you live
- affordability

Deciding on a treatment plan that is *right* for you

At the beginning of this book I described some medical problems that can cause or worsen symptoms of MCI and dementia including vascular diseases that affect the arteries of the brain, Parkinson's disease and other progressive neurodegenerative disorders, traumatic brain injury (TBI), HIV/AIDS, cerebrovascular accidents (i.e. stroke), and the cumulative toxic effects of chronic alcohol or drug abuse.

In contrast to neurodegenerative disorders and other irreversible causes of dementia, when an underlying medical problem is diagnosed and properly treated, mild to moderate symptoms of memory loss, confusion or other symptoms of cognitive impairment (i.e., delirium) may improve rapidly, and a treatment you—or someone you are caring for—have been taking may start to work better.

If you—or a person you are caring for—are experiencing symptoms of severe cognitive impairment, or if you think you have a medical problem that may be causing your memory problem or making it worse, *I encourage you to seek medical care before starting any new treatment including those discussed in this book.*

First steps

Since you've gotten this far, I am assuming that you—or someone you are caring for—*don't' have a medical problem* that is causing memory loss, confusion or other symptoms of cognitive impairment. If this is the case, you're ready to start working on a holistic treatment plan that addresses your particular symptoms keeping in mind approaches that are available where you live and affordable.

This section will guide you through the steps needed to develop an appropriate treatment plan whether you—or someone you are caring for—have mild, moderate or severe symptoms of memory loss or other symptoms of cognitive impairment. The first step in deciding on an appropriate treatment plan involves identifying one or more treatments that you—or a person you are caring for—are *open to* trying.

When deciding on a treatment plan you probably have a better chance of *functioning better* if you use at least one tier A treatment. Although some currently available mainstream and alternative treatments of MCI and dementia slow the rate of cognitive decline, *no existing treatments stop progressive cognitive decline or reverse the causes of dementia.*

At this time, Tier A alternative treatments of MCI and dementia with established efficacy for slowing the rate of progression of cognitive decline are:

- dietary change

- regular exercise

- a standardized extract of the herbal *Ginkgo biloba*

- Idebenone, a semi-synthetic derivative of a natural supplement

I encourage you to start with one or more Tier A treatments if you—or someone you are caring for—have severe cognitive problems that are impairing your ability to function day to day. In addition to alternative treatment approaches you may also need to take *a cholinesterase inhibitor or other medication*.

Even if you are taking a medication, you may benefit from taking one or more natural supplements (*but only after confirming it is safe to do so*) or trying some of the other approaches described in this book. In addition to *Ginkgo biloba* and idebenone, other natural supplements reviewed in this book may provide temporary relief from—or slow the rate of progression of—mild to moderate symptoms of memory loss or other cognitive problems. Most supplements reviewed in this book may be safely combined with medications used to treat MCI and dementia, in some cases increasing their effectiveness (please see comments on *adverse effects and warnings* under the supplement that interests you).

Besides natural supplements, other alternative approaches that may temporarily mitigate the cognitive and behavioral symptoms of MCI and dementia, or slow the rate of progression of cognitive decline include regular exercise, the practice of Tai Chi or Qigong, bright light exposure therapy, Healing Touch, listening to soothing music, access to wander gardens, transcranial electrical stimulation, multi-modality treatment protocols. and transcranial low-level laser therapy (TLLLT).

If you—or a person you are caring for—are currently taking a medication for symptoms of MCI or dementia, I strongly encourage you to *seek advice from a psychiatrist before starting any other medication or a natural supplement.*

Taking care of mild or early symptoms of MCI and dementia

If you are experiencing mild or moderate symptoms of memory loss or other problems with cognitive functioning, you may benefit from adopting a Mediterranean diet, moderating alcohol consumption, and engaging in more frequent physical activity. In addition to making life style changes, natural supplements and mind-body approaches can sometimes help improve memory and global cognitive functioning. For example, taking a standardized formula of *Ginkgo biloba*, acetyl-l-carnitine, a combination of vitamins C and E, or engaging in a regular mind-body practice such as Tai Chi or Qigong may improve your memory and your overall level of cognitive functioning.

Multi-modality approaches such as the Bredesen protocol incorporate a variety of approaches including dietary changes, natural supplements, sleep hygiene, regular exercise and other lifestyle modifications with the goal of slowing down and possibly reversing MCI and Alzheimer's disease. Although multi-modality approaches have not been substantiated by large controlled studies, several carefully documented case reports suggest that strict adherence to such protocols over several months can result in dramatic improvement in cognitive functioning in individuals with MCI or early stages of Alzheimer's disease.

Even if you have already tried tier A approaches without success, you may benefit from a tier B or tier C approach. For example, tier B treatments such as folate, thiamin and vitamin B-12, the herbal huperzine, some compound herbal formulas used in Asian medicine and acetyl-l-carnitine, may improve memory and cognitive functioning, in some cases permitting a reduction in the dose of a cholinesterase inhibitor or other prescription medication. Emerging research findings support that that a compound herbal formula called SLT may significantly reduce the severity of cognitive impairment caused by vascular dementia.

Even if you've already tried different approaches listed in Tiers A and B with little or no benefit, you may benefit from one or more Tier C therapies. Although treatments listed in Tier C are supported by less evidence than Tier A and B approaches, preliminary research findings for some are very promising. For example, multi-modality protocols and transcranial photobiomodulation are currently listed in Tier C because of the paucity of research evidence supporting their use as treatments of MCI and dementia. However, preliminary findings suggest that both approaches are effective and may soon emerge as mainstream treatments. If future studies confirm early findings of dramatic improvement in symptoms of MCI and dementia, these and possibly other treatment approaches currently included in Tier C may move to Tier B or Tier A.

Before trying a Tier B treatment or a combination of treatments from Tier A and Tier B, I encourage you to first carefully review the detailed descriptions of treatments you've already tried to *be sure you've used them in ways and for durations that are expected to be* effective.

Some people who have used a particular natural supplement with disappointing results find out later that they had been taking a dosage that was too low, stopped taking it before it had enough time to work, or were not using a quality brand. I encourage you to check the on-line resources at the end of this book to compare different brands of the natural supplement you've already tried. *If it turns out you didn't take a Tier A or B treatment at the recommended dosage or you used a brand of poor or uncertain quality, I encourage you to try the same treatment again, this time taking a quality brand at the recommended dosage and for the recommended duration.*

The above reasoning applies equally to treatments other than natural supplements. For example, if you previously tried a mind-body therapy (e.g., Tai Chi or Qigong) or an energy therapy (e.g., transcranial electrical stimulation, bright light exposure therapy or low level laser therapy), and your response was disappointing I encourage you to check the information in the treatment summaries before concluding that a particular mind-body or energy treatment is *not* beneficial.

If you were not working with an experienced practitioner when you previously tried a mind-body approach, you may not have used the most effective technique or tried the approach for an amount of time that would be expected to consistently improve your memory or other areas of cognitive functioning. In that case, I encourage you to first re-evaluate the way you previously used the mind-body practice or energy therapy to find out whether you were doing so in a way that would be expected to be beneficial.

Other considerations

In addition to alternative treatment preferences you have after reading this book, I encourage you to remain open to other approaches before deciding on a final treatment plan. If you've already tried several different treatments one at a time, you may have more success trying two or more approaches at the same time starting with treatments in Tiers A and B. This strategy can be especially helpful if:

- you've already tried most or all treatments listed in Tier A and they haven't helped
- a Tier A treatment you've previously tried was helpful but caused side effects and you had to stop using it
- There is evidence that combining a particular Tier B or C treatment with a particular Tier A treatment will work better than taking a Tier A treatment alone
- a preferred Tier A treatment is unavailable where you live or too expensive

When to self-treat memory loss and when to seek advice from a psychiatrist or other healthcare provider

After you have identified approaches you would like to try, the next step involves deciding whether to follow your treatment plan on your own or see a psychiatrist or other healthcare provider for expert advice and guidance. The information included under the various treatments will help you decide between self-care and working with a healthcare provider. I encourage you to consult with a psychiatrist if you are experiencing severe memory loss or other severe cognitive problems (e.g. confusion, frequently getting lost in familiar places) or *if you are considering taking any natural supplement together with a medication.*

Below I've listed some important points that will help you find an experienced alternative healthcare practitioner:

- A physician or other conventional healthcare provider you already know can often help you find an experienced practitioner of an alternative therapy that interests you. You can probably get helpful information about local alternative practitioners from a clinic near you. Many alternative healthcare practitioners are members of a professional association of certified practitioners in their field. A representative of the appropriate professional association—whether it is for practitioners of Chinese medicine, herbal medicine, yoga, or any another healing discipline—can probably recommend one or more practitioners near you.

- Once you've identified a practitioner of a therapy that interests you, I encourage you to learn everything you can about their background, including their education, training, licensing, and any advanced certifications. Different professional groups and different countries impose a wide variety of requirements on health care providers in terms of training and standards of practice. The most important thing is to identify a practitioner who has a good reputation among his or her colleagues and has a great deal of experience treating individuals struggling with MCI or dementia.

- The next step involves finding out what the treatment costs. I am assuming that many readers have health insurance which may cover at least part of the cost of treatment. Not checking on cost and insurance issues before starting treatment can result in an expensive and brief encounter with even the most qualified mainstream or alternative practitioner, and leave you feeling disappointed and frustrated with fewer resources remaining to help you get the care you need.

- At the first session it is important to provide your new health care provider with a complete list of mainstream and alternative treatments you've already tried including those that did not work or caused side effects. Your new provider will use this information to identify approaches that are more likely to be beneficial while minimizing the risk of side effects.

- Be sure to tell your new health care provider *and all other providers*, about changes in your symptoms, any new medical problems, and new treatments that you decide to try. Good communication between yourself and your health care providers will ensure they have the information they need to give you the best possible care.

Safety is *always* the *Number 1* priority

Safety is the *single most important consideration* when thinking of starting any new treatment—including a medication, a natural supplement—or a combination of two or more different treatments. I've included important safety information under all supplements so that you can review this material before starting a natural supplement or taking it in combination with another supplement or a medication.

I encourage you to work with a psychiatrist or other medically trained provider *when considering taking any natural supplement together with any medication*. Though serious safety problems are uncommon, *combinations of certain supplements and medications can result in toxic interactions that may be dangerous and in rare cases life-threatening.*

In the treatment summaries I list established safety concerns for natural supplements when taken alone or together with medications. There is a great deal to know about safety that I cannot adequately cover in this short book. **Before taking any natural supplement together with a medication I encourage you to check the on-line resources at the end of this book to find out whether the specific combination you are considering is both safe and effective.**

Making changes along the way: re-evaluating the treatment plan and making it better

This section will help you find out how well your treatment plan is working and know what to do if it is not helping. You will learn when to continue the current treatment plan, change it, or stop it all together.

If you—or a person you are caring for—are not functioning consistently better *after following the initial treatment plan for the suggested amount of time* it is important re-evaluate what you are doing and consider making changes. If there is evidence that a medical problem may be causing memory loss or confusion, or interfering with treatment, I encourage you to see a psychiatrist or other medically trained provider to make sure the problem is not making your memory problem worse or interfering with the beneficial effects of treatment.

If the treatment plan involves taking a natural supplement or using another approach supported by solid evidence, and you—or a person you are caring for—have followed the plan for the *amount of time usually needed to achieve beneficial results but there has been little or no improvement in cognitive functioning*, it is reasonable to consider several options including:

- Increasing the dosage of a natural supplement or medication

- Finding a higher quality brand of a natural supplement or medication

- Increasing the frequency of a whole-body, mind-body or energy therapy

- Adding another approach to your existing treatment plan

- Switching to an entirely new treatment plan

- Stopping treatment all together

If you've already tried several approaches in tiers A and B but without success, you may benefit from combining a tier A and tier B treatment, two tier A treatments, or two treatments from tier B—*assuming it is safe to do so*. Although tier C treatments are supported by less evidence than tier A and B treatments, many people benefit from tier C treatments.

New research findings are constantly being reported at conferences and in medical journals showing that some treatments supported by weak or inconclusive research findings in the journal literature may actually be more effective than previously believed.

The amount of time it takes to function consistently better after starting any treatment or treatment combination, depends on many factors including how severe your memory loss or other symptoms of cognitive impairment are, the particular treatment of treatments you are using, the amount of stress you are under, your general state of health and how closely you've been following your plan.

Most medications and supplements take time to work so it may take several weeks to experience consistent improvement in memory or other areas of cognitive functioning after starting a new medication or natural supplement. Information on how much time it usually takes for particular alternative treatments to work is included in the treatment summaries.

Deciding when to change your treatment plan

The following questions will help you decide when to think about changing your treatment plan.

How do I know if my current treatment plan is working?

If you are functioning better most of the time your current treatment plan is probably working well. On the other hand, if forgetfulness or other cognitive problems have not improved since starting treatment, your current plan clearly isn't working, or you may not be using a particular treatment in the most effective way.

Some people take longer than others to respond to the same dose of a particular medication, natural supplement or the same level of commitment to a mind-body practice, dietary changes or exercise. If your current treatment plan is improving your memory and you are functioning better at work, in a relationship or other aspects of your life but you—or a person you are caring for—continue to struggle with forgetfulness, confusion or other cognitive problems, you may benefit from adjusting dosages (of a medication or natural supplement) or increasing the frequency of workouts, a mind-body practice or another approach you've been trying, while continuing to follow the same general treatment plan as before.

It is important to make decisions about changing or stopping your treatment plan on the basis of an accurate assessment of your symptoms. For this reason, I encourage you to answer the questions in the same [self-assessment inventory](#) you used when deciding on your initial treatment plan. The results will help you to find out whether your symptoms are the same, worse or better than before.

Taking inventory of symptoms will give you the information you need to decide whether to continue your current treatment plan, try something new, or stop treatment all together. Keeping a record of your answers will provide useful information about changes in your symptoms over time and which treatments are more effective.

If I'm not functioning better how much longer should I wait before considering starting a new treatment?

The answer to this question depends on many factors that are different for each person. The amount of time needed to achieve consistent improvement in memory or other problems in cognitive functioning in response to a particular treatment is listed under that treatment (i.e., when known). In general, if a treatment you—or a person you are caring for—are using now worked in the past it will probably be effective this time. Unless you have severe memory loss that is impairing your ability to work, be in a relationship or function in other areas of your life, or you are experiencing serious side effects to a medication or natural supplement, I encourage you to continue your current treatment plan for several more weeks before trying something new.

How concerned should I be about side effects and what can I do if I get them? Making decisions about changing your treatment plan based on side effects has to do with how serious they are and how much they interfere with your ability to function day to day. If you have mild side effects caused by a medication or a natural supplement that don't impair your ability to work or function in other ways your body may *get used* to these side effects fairly soon. On the other hand, if you—or a person you are caring for—are having side effects that interfere with daily activities it is prudent to stop your current treatment plan and try something new.

Depending on the medication or natural supplement that is causing side effects, changing the dosage or adding another medication or supplement can sometimes reduce or completely eliminate the problem. Of course, adding another medication or natural supplement may also cause new side effects. Before making any changes in your treatment plan aimed at reducing side effects, I encourage you to get expert advice from a psychiatrist or other medically trained provider.

When should I try something new in addition to my current treatment? How do I decide what to try next?

As a general rule it is best to keep your treatment plan as simple as possible and avoid combinations of treatments that cause potentially serious safety problems. If you are functioning better on your current treatment plan and your memory loss or other cognitive problems aren't severe, I encourage you to wait a little longer before trying something new. On the other hand, if you aren't functioning consistently better on your current treatment, or you are experiencing severe memory loss, daily confusion or other symptoms of severe cognitive impairment, I encourage you to consider trying something new that may enhance the beneficial effects of your current treatment.

Deciding whether to add a new treatment to your ongoing treatment plan depends on the likelihood that the change will result in improvements in cognitive functioning that would otherwise not take place. Deciding whether to add another treatment to your current plan also depends on whether the potential risk of side effects outweighs the potential benefits of starting a new treatment.

Before deciding whether to try two or more treatments at the same time I encourage you to first review the information in the treatment summaries to learn about specific combinations known to be *synergistic and safe*. In order to minimize the risk of side effects and potentially unsafe interactions please exercise caution when adding any new treatment to an existing treatment—whether it is a medication, a natural supplement or something else.

When should I stop what I'm taking and try something new or take no treatment at all?

If you are following your current treatment plan taking a quality brand natural product or medication at the recommended dosage, or using a mind-body or energy therapy on a regular basis but you are not functioning consistently better, it may be time to discontinue your current treatment plan and wait before starting any new treatment. For example, if you are taking a medication or a natural supplement under the advice of a physician or alternative medical practitioner, I encourage you to see your provider for advice on how to safely discontinue the medication (or supplement) before starting any new treatment.

For the most part, gradually decreasing the dosage of a medication or supplement reduces the risk of side effects that can take place when abruptly stopping a treatment. In some cases, especially for less severe memory loss or other mild symptoms of cognitive impairment, you may function and feel better after stopping a medication or a natural supplement.

If you have been diagnosed with MCI or are in the early stages of Alzheimer's disease, maintaining a healthy life style including regular exercise, following a Mediterranean diet, getting enough sleep, and following a regular stress management program, may improve your memory and reduce the severity of other cognitive problems, even in the absence of treatment. However, if you—or a person you are caring for—are impaired by severe memory loss or other severe cognitive problems, it is prudent to consider adding another treatment to boost the effectiveness of the current treatment, or to consider switching to an entirely new treatment.

Before doing either of these, I encourage you to first consult with a psychiatrist or other medically trained provider for expert advice and guidance. When deciding whether to try any new treatment for MCI or dementia use the same steps you followed when developing the initial treatment plan.

When should I see a psychiatrist or other health care provider for expert advice including questions about dosages, concerns about adverse effects, or to find out whether I have a medical problem?

It is prudent to consult with a psychiatrist or other health care provider if you—or a person you are caring for—are experiencing side effects caused by a medication or a natural supplement. I also encourage you to see a psychiatrist or other medically trained provider if you think you have a medical problem in order to get a thorough evaluation and to find out whether your medical problem is causing memory loss, confusion or other cognitive symptoms, making your situation worse or interfering with your response to treatment.

Repeating the steps until you find a treatment plan that *works* *for you*

Sometimes it is necessary to try many different approaches in order to get to a treatment plan that works. Every time you go through the process of deciding on a treatment plan you will have a better understanding of the nature and severity of your memory problem (or other cognitive problems) and how your symptoms change over time. You will also have useful insights about treatments that work as well as ones that *don't work.*

When evaluating your memory problem, you can use the same self-assessment questionnaire as many times as you need to. By saving your answers you can track how your symptoms respond to changes in your treatment plan. This information will help you decide whether to continue on your current treatment, try something new or stop treatment all together.

If you have not experienced consistent improvement in your memory or other cognitive problems, after trying two different treatment plans, I encourage you to seek advice from a psychiatrist or other medically trained provider.

Finally—and I can't emphasize this point strongly enough—if in addition to your memory problem you are severely depressed or have another serious mental health problem, or if you think you have a medical problem that may be causing your memory loss or making it worse, I encourage you to seek immediate medical care.

Summary of main points

Below I summarize the most important points in this book including key steps involved in developing a safe, effective and affordable treatment plan for MCI or dementia based on your history, symptoms, preferences and circumstances:

- *If you—or someone you are caring for—are experiencing severe memory loss or other severe symptoms of cognitive impairment, or if you think you have a medical or mental health problem that may be causing memory loss, confusion or impairing your ability to function, I urge you to seek urgent care at the nearest hospital or emergency room.*
- This book is offered as a practical resource on *alternative* treatments of mild cognitive impairment (MCI) and dementia.
- Alternative medicine sometimes called 'complementary and alternative medicine or CAM—consists of approaches that are currently not used in mainstream Western medicine (also called 'biomedicine' and 'allopathic medicine').
- Integrative medicine is a person-centered approach to care that incorporates mainstream Western medical treatments and CAM approaches.

- Integrative mental health care is the area of integrative medicine aimed at optimizing emotional and mental wellness and treating specific mental health problems.
- If you—or a person you are caring for—have recently been hospitalized or evaluated in an emergency room for a severe memory problem, confusion or other symptoms of impaired cognitive functioning, and you are functioning better now, this book will help you identify appropriate alternative treatment approaches.
- If you think you—or a person you are caring for—may have a medical problem that has not been diagnosed, is not being properly treated, or has recently been getting worse, I encourage you to see a physician or other medically trained provider before making *any* changes in your current treatment plan or starting any new treatment. A large number of medical problems can cause temporary disruption of normal cognitive functioning manifesting as delirium with memory loss, confusion and other problems.

The type and severity of cognitive symptoms are related to the underlying causes of delirium.

- With proper treatment of delirium normal brain function is restored and cognitive problems often resolve rapidly and completely. However, as many as 1/3 of individuals diagnosed with MCI eventually progress to full-blown dementia, thus MCI may represent the early phase of progressive deterioration in cognitive functioning that leads to Alzheimer's disease or another type of dementia. Medical problems that can cause dementia include vascular disease that affects the arteries of the brain, Parkinson's disease, other neurodegenerative disorders, traumatic brain injury (TBI), HIV/AIDS, severe cerebrovascular accidents (i.e. stroke), and the cumulative toxic effects of chronic alcohol or substance abuse.
- The first step in developing an appropriate treatment plan involves *taking inventory of your* symptoms using the self-assessment questionnaires provided on the companion

[website](). Your answers will help you better understand the nature and severity of your memory problem, confusion or other cognitive symptoms.

- After taking inventory of your symptoms, the next step is to carefully review the evidence for various treatments and to identify those treatments that make sense in view of your history and symptoms.

- The next step involves deciding whether to start treatment on your own or to work with a psychiatrist or other medically trained provider.

- Mild to moderately severe memory loss in MCI or the early stages of Alzheimer's disease, may respond to changes in life style such as regular exercise and adherence to a Mediterranean diet.

- Severe symptoms of cognitive impairment seldom respond to life style changes alone, may be related to an underlying medical problem or a progressive neurodegenerative disorder, and may require long-term treatment with a medication, a natural supplement, or a medication and a natural supplement in combination. Decisions about combining any two or more medications or supplements should be based on scientific evidence and safety considerations. ***If you are experiencing severe memory loss, confusion or other symptoms of severe, persistent or progressively worsening cognitive impairment, I strongly encourage you work closely with a psychiatrist or other medically trained provider who can evaluate you and advise you on the most appropriate treatment for you.***

- Even if you—or a person you are caring for—need a medication or a natural supplement in order to function consistently better, making positive lifestyle changes such as exercising more often, adhering to a Mediterranean diet, and a daily mind-body practice, may improve your memory and your overall level of cognitive functioning.

- When deciding on a treatment plan first consider tier A treatments supported by strong evidence. If you have already tried treatments in tier A—but without benefit, I encourage you to review the detailed information in this book on those treatments you've tried to make sure you used a quality brand (i.e. if it is a natural supplement) at the recommended dosage and for the recommended period of time. By the same token, if you've been following a Mediterranean diet or exercising on a regular basis, but your memory loss or other cognitive problems haven't improved, I encourage you to review the information on both approaches to make sure you are modifying your diet in ways that would be expected to help, and exercising in a way and for a duration that would be expected to improve your memory or your general cognitive functioning.

- If after reviewing the bullets under treatments you've previously tried you discover that you did not try a particular tier A or B treatment at the optimal dosage and for a duration that would be expected to result in improved cognitive functioning, I encourage you to try that treatment again. This time make sure you use the recommended dosage of a quality brand for the recommended amount of time. By the same token, if you previously tried a whole body, mind-body or energetic approach known to be beneficial for memory loss or other cognitive problems, but without benefit, I encourage you to try that approach again, this time closely following recommendations on frequency and duration of treatment that would most likely achieve beneficial results.

- An important consideration is deciding whether to try one treatment or a combination or two or more treatments at the same time. *Examples of beneficial combinations as well as unsafe combinations to be avoided* are included in the detailed information under the various treatments.

- If symptoms of forgetfulness, or another cognitive problem are not responding to the initial treatment plan *after following it for the recommended amount of time,* I encourage you to find a psychiatrist or other medically trained health care provider to obtain diagnostic tests in order to make sure that a medical problem is not causing your memory problem, making it worse, or interfering your response to treatment.
- If your memory loss or other cognitive problems do not improve after you've followed your treatment plan for a period of time after which you should expect results, I encourage you to consider switching to a different treatment, preferably one that belongs to tier A or tier B. Again, the amount of time in which you should expect improvement in response to a particular treatment is discussed under each treatment (i.e., when known). Depending on the severity of your symptoms, it may be

helpful to continue your current treatment while adding one or more new approaches.

- Make sure you know about safety concerns associated with any treatment or treatment combinations you are considering. Safety problems are described under the specific treatments. *Before combining two or more treatments first review the comments on safe and effective treatment combinations as well as warnings pertaining to particular treatment combinations. It is always best to avoid combining two or more treatments that can potentially result in a toxic interaction.* If you decide to combine two or more treatments after reviewing the information in this book, I encourage you to first consult with a psychiatrist or other medically trained provider for expert advice and guidance.

- From time to time it is important to take a close look at your memory problem or other cognitive problems—*even when your treatment plan is working well.* Taking a self-inventory by answering standardized questions will help you understand your symptoms better and determine whether you are experiencing significant new symptoms of memory loss, confusion or another mental health problem.

- Continue to modify your treatment plan on an on-going basis using an appropriate self-assessment inventory to document any changes in symptoms. Changes in the type or severity of your symptoms may call for changes in the treatment plan. If you are not functioning consistently better after trying at least two different treatment plans for the recommended period of time please seek professional care for formal evaluation and expert advice.

- If you are experiencing moderately severe memory loss, confusion or other cognitive problems after trying at least two separate treatment approaches, you may be able to remain at your current level of functioning after discontinuing treatment. Some people who have moderately severe memory loss benefit from life-style changes such as regular exercise, improved nutrition, and stress management.

Going deeper

After reading this book on alternative treatments of dementia and mild cognitive impairment you may want to learn more. You can find in-depth information in my other books:

- *An Integrative Paradigm for Mental Health Care: Ideas and Methods Shaping the Future*, Springer, 2019

- *Textbook of Integrative Mental Health Care*, Thieme Medical, 2006

- *Integrative Mental Health Care: A Therapist's Handbook*, Norton 2009

- *Complementary and Alternative Treatments in Mental Health Care*, American Psychiatric Association, Inc. 2006

- *Chinese Medical Psychiatry: A Textbook and Clinical Manual*, Blue Poppy Press, 2000

You can find links to all of my books, as well as many full-text articles and conference presentations on my website http://progressivepsychiatry.com/

Finding quality products and services on the Internet

After you've decided on the treatment plan that makes sense for you the next step is to find quality products and services that you can use. This section includes valuable internet resources that will help you select safe, effective and affordable products and services. Some of the resources listed are free while others charge a subscription fee.

General resources on complementary and alternative treatment approaches

- **Progressive Psychiatry** http://progressivepsychiatry.com/ This is the author's website. It includes a comprehensive list of on-line resources on both mainstream mental health care and complementary and alternative medicine (CAM) approaches. You can find several full-text articles published by Dr. Lake as well as presentations made at various conferences over the years. The site also includes a blog on integrative mental health care and links to all of Dr. Lake's books.

- **The National Center for Complementary and Integrative Health (NCCIH)** https://nccih.nih.gov is part of the National Institutes of Health (NIH). NCCIH is dedicated to exploring complementary and alternative healing practices in the context of rigorous science, training complementary and alternative medicine (CAM) researchers, and disseminating authoritative information to the public and professionals. The site contains extensive reviews of research on all non-medication treatment approaches. A citation index contains over 200,000 citations of studies on all areas of non-conventional medicine indexed in the National Library of Medicine beginning in 1966. The section includes valuable advice on how to find qualified practitioners of alternative and integrative medicine. The site includes information **en Español.**

Resources on dietary supplements (no fee)

- **National Institutes of Health Office of Dietary Supplements** https://ods.od.nih.gov/ provides an extensive on-line library of dietary supplement fact sheets for widely used herbals and other natural products. Different versions are available for consumers and health professionals. The site includes frequently asked questions (FAQs) and links to scientific monographs. The site includes some information **en Español.**

- **Medline Plus Supplement Information** https://medlineplus.gov/druginformation.html is a service of the U.S. National Library of Medicine, National Institutes of Health. It includes a comprehensive library of on-line monographs on prescription drugs as well as herbals and other natural product supplements. Each monograph includes safety information on adverse effects and interactions. The site also includes free mental health screening tools, educational brochures, videos and podcasts on common mental health problems.

- **Drugs.com** https://www.drugs.com/ includes a comprehensive library of on-line monographs on prescription medications and natural products including extensive information on adverse effects. It includes an on-line tool for checking interactions. Different versions are available for consumers and health professionals. The information on the site is also available **en Español**.

- **National Herbalists Association of Australia** https://www.nhaa.org.au Founded in 1920, the National Herbalists Association of Australia is the oldest natural therapies association in Australia, and the only national professional body of medical herbalists. Their mission is to serve and support membership (Medical Herbalists and Naturopaths) and to promote and protect the profession and practice of herbal medicine. This website is a portal to on-line resources covering all aspects of herbal medicine as well as complementary and alternative medicine in general. It includes links to valuable resources on research, nutrition, herbals and other natural product supplements, professional associations, educational resources, and reputable distributors and suppliers of herbals and other natural products.

- **The World Health Organization's (WHO) traditional medicine portal** https://www.who.int/traditional-complementary-integrative-medicine/en/ provides a traditional medicine fact sheet and links to worldwide health care resources. WHO seeks to promote international collaboration and cooperation in the study and use of traditional healing approaches in mental health care.

Resources on natural products and other non-medication treatments (fee)

- **ConsumerLab.com** https://www.consumerlab.com/ provides independent test results and information to help consumers and healthcare professionals evaluate health, wellness, and nutrition products. ConsumerLab is a certification company and enables companies of all sizes to have their products voluntarily tested for potential inclusion in its list of Approved Quality products and bear its seal of approval. The site is a valuable consumer resource for evaluating different natural products and brands and identifying brands that are both safe and effective.

- **Natural Medicines** https://naturalmedicines.therapeuticresearch.com is a subscription service that provides valuable information on natural products and other non-medication approaches. Like Consumerlab.com, Natural Medicines provides independent reviews of supplements that are authoritative and easy to read. The site provides links to valuable databases on natural products and other approaches. It also includes consumer monographs, patient handouts and offers continuing education credit on different topics to health professionals.

- **Herb Research Foundation** http://www.herbs.org/hrfinfo.html includes expert compilations on specific herbals that contain carefully selected articles, studies, and discussions by experts that are available as downloads or in print form. The work of the Herb Research Foundation is based on its dedicated holdings of more than 300,000 scientific articles on thousands of herbs.

www.ingramcontent.com/pod-product-compliance
Lightning Source LLC
Chambersburg PA
CBHW030651220526
45463CB00005B/1724